Copyright © 2022 by Martina Giokos, RDN

Table of Contents

When shopping at the grocery store, the foods you grab can greatly impact your overall health. In fact, filling your cart with a lot of refined grains, sugary drinks, and processed foods can increase inflammation and affect your health.

Therefore, filling up on healthy foods can help keep you healthy, protect against chronic diseases resistant to drugs and rid your body of toxins.

We also absorb tons of toxins every day through the air we breathe, the water we drink, the food we eat, and by just being outside in our surroundings.

So how do we get rid of these toxins that can be harmful to our body? It's through the Healing diet.

The Healing foods diet is not just a diet; It is a tool that will lead you to a total transformation of your health. This diet was designed to help everyone overcome diseases. It is designed to heal your body and improve your health by encouraging the consumption of nutritious, whole foods like fruits, veggies, legumes, healthy fats, organic meats, and healing herbs and spices.

Plus, this simple eating pattern is a great way to ensure you supply your body with a steady stream of the nutrients you need to help prevent nutritional deficiencies in your diet and to promote healthy living.

So what makes this diet unique?

This diet is unique because it involves making some simple switches in your diet compared to other complicated diets with many rules and regulations.

1. Cranberry and Orange Balls

Prep: 50 mins

Total: 50 mins

Servings: 15

Ingredients

- 12 medjool dates, pitted
- 1 tbsp honey
- 2 tsp finely grated orange rind
- 1/2 cup cashew spread
- 1/2 cup LSA (linseed, sunflower seeds and almonds)
- 1/4 cup shredded coconut
- 1/4 cup dried cranberries
- 3/4 cup pistachio kernels, toasted

Directions

1. Place dates, honey, orange rind, cashew spread, LSA, coconut, cranberries and 1/4 cup pistachios in a food processor.
2. Process until well combined and a coarse mixture forms.
3. Finely chop remaining pistachios. Place in a small bowl.
4. Press and roll level tablespoons of mixture into balls. Roll in pistachios to lightly coat. Place balls on a plate. Refrigerate for 20 minutes or until firm. Serve.

Prep: 10 mins

Cook: 15 mins

Total: 25 mins

Servings: 4

Ingredients

- 1 large (about 1.2kg) cauliflower
- 1/4 cup extra virgin olive oil, plus extra for frying
- 1 tsp ground turmeric
- Fried curry leaves, to serve
- Thinly sliced fried red chilli, to serve

Directions

1. Preheat oven to 180 degrees C/160 degrees C fan forced. Line 2 baking trays with foil.
2. Cut the cauliflower into four 1.5cm-thick slices, leaving base intact. Cook steaks in extra virgin

olive oil in a non-stick frying pan over medium-high heat for 2-3 minutes each side or until golden. Transfer to the foil-lined baking tray.

3. Whisk the olive oil with the turmeric in a bowl until combined. Brush over steaks.

4. Roast cauliflower in the oven for 12-15 minutes or until tender and crisp.

5. Scatter with fried curry leaves and thinly sliced red chilli, to serve.

3. Curried Lentil Soup

Prep: 10 mins

Cook: 20 mins

Total: 30 mins

Servings: 6

Ingredients

- medium white onion, diced (approx. 2 cups, 300 g)
- 3 carrots, chopped into thick rounds (approx. 2 cups, 300 g)
- 3 cloves garlic, minced
- 3 stalks celery, chopped (approx. 320 g)
- 1 tbsp curry powder
- 1 tsp each cumin and coriander
- 1/2 tsp each salt and pepper
- 1 1/2 cups uncooked red lentils
- 1 14 oz can light coconut milk
- 1 28 oz can diced tomatoes with the juices

- 4 cups vegetable stock
- 1 tbsp soy sauce or gluten-free tamari
- 1 tsp coconut sugar or pure maple syrup

Directions

1. Add the carrots, celery, onion and garlic to a soup pot with 2 tbsp water or broth. Cook over medium heat, stirring often, for 5-6 minutes.
2. Add the spices and stir to combine. Cook for another minute or two, adding 1-2 tbsp more water or broth if the pot is getting too dry.
3. Add the lentils, diced tomatoes, coconut milk and broth and stir to combine.
4. Simmer for 20-25 minutes, uncovered over low to medium heat until the lentils are soft and almost mushy.
5. Stir in the coconut sugar and soy sauce (or gluten-free tamari).
6. Serve right away topped with fresh cilantro, if desired.

Prep: 15 mins

Cook: 25 mins

Total: 40 mins

Servings: 4

Ingredients

- 1 cup (200g) pearl barley
- 250g broccoli, cut into small florets
- 100g green beans, trimmed, halved lengthways
- 1/2 cup (60g) frozen peas
- 1 lemon, sliced
- 10cm-piece ginger, grated
- 2 tbsp soy sauce
- 4 skinless salmon fillets
- 1/2 baby cos lettuce, leaves, torn
- 1 small red onion, cut into rings
- 1 tsp grated ginger, extra
- 2 spring onions, thinly sliced

- 1 tbsp rice wine vinegar
- 1 tbsp extra virgin olive oil

Directions

1. Cook barley in a large saucepan of salted boiling water for 25 mins or until tender, adding broccoli during the last 5 mins and the beans and peas during last 2 mins of cooking time. Rinse under cold water. Drain.

2. Meanwhile, place lemon, ginger and 3 cups (750ml) water in a large frying pan over medium heat. Bring to a simmer. Reduce heat to low. Add salmon. Cook for 8 mins or until cooked to your liking. Remove salmon from poaching liquid. Flake into large pieces.
Combine barley, broccoli mixture, salmon, lettuce and onion in a large bowl. Whisk extra ginger, spring onion, vinegar and oil in a small bowl. Add to salmon mixture, toss to combine. Serve.

Prep: 5 mins

Cook: 8 hrs

Total: 8 hrs 5 mins

Servings: 4

Ingredients

- 150g (1 cup) steel cut oats
- 875ml (3 1/2 cups) water
- 1 large red apple, peeled and coarsely grated
- 1 tsp vanilla extract
- 1 cinnamon stick
- Yoghurt, to serve
- Sliced apple, to serve
- Fresh raspberries, to serve
- Toasted nuts and seeds, to serve
- Maple syrup, to serve

Directions

1. Lightly grease a 3L slow-cooker with oil. Add the oats, water, apple and vanilla. Stir to combine then add the cinnamon stick.

2. Set the slow-cooker on low and cook for 8 hours. Remove and discard cinnamon stick and stir well. Stand uncovered for 5 minutes.

3. Serve with a dollop of yoghurt, sprinkled with apple, nuts and seeds and drizzled with maple syrup.

Prep: 5 mins

Cook: 5 mins

Total: 10 mins

Servings: 1

Ingredients

- 2 slices wholemeal sourdough bread, toasted
- 2 tsp nut butter
- Pinch of ground cinnamon
- 1/2 banana, sliced
- 1/4 cup fresh blueberries

Directions

1. Spread toast with nut butter.
2. Top with banana and blueberries.
3. Sprinkle with cinnamon.

Prep: 10 mins

Total: 10 mins

Servings: 4

Ingredients

- 2 tablespoons extra-virgin olive oil
- 2 tablespoons fresh lemon juice
- 1 tablespoon chopped fresh oregano
- 4 cups (packed) baby spinach leaves, coarsely chopped (about 4 ounces)
- 1 1/2 large red bell peppers, diced
- 1 1/2 cups diced celery (about 3 stalks)
- 3/4 cup crumbled soft fresh goat cheese
- 1/3 cup chopped red onion

Directions

1. Whisk oil, lemon juice, and oregano in large bowl to blend.
2. Season to taste with salt and pepper. Add spinach, bell peppers, celery, goat cheese, and red onion to dressing; toss to coat.
3. Divide salad among 4 plates and serve.

Prep: 15 mins

Cook: 10 mins

Total: 25 mins

Servings: 4

Ingredients

- 2 large heads (700g) broccoli, chopped
- 2 tbsp gluten-free cornflour
- 1/2 tsp dried red chilli flakes
- 1/2 tsp turmeric
- 250g firm tofu, drained, cut into 1cm pieces
- 1 tbsp macadamia oil
- 2 garlic cloves, crushed
- 2 large carrots, peeled, cut into thin matchsticks
- 4 green shallots, thinly sliced, plus extra, to serve
- 1 large red capsicum, deseeded, thinly sliced
- 1 tbsp salt-reduced gluten-free tamari

- 1/3 cup fresh coriander leaves, plus extra, to serve
- 1 tbsp sunflower seeds, toasted

Directions

1. Process the broccoli in a food processor, in 2 batches, until it is finely chopped and resembles grains of rice. Set aside.
2. Combine the cornflour, chilli flakes and turmeric in a snap-lock bag. Add the tofu. Seal the bag and toss until tofu is coated. Shake off any excess corn flour mixture.
3. Heat half the oil in a large wok over high heat. Stir-fry tofu in 2 batches, for 2 minutes or until golden. Transfer to a plate.
4. Heat the remaining oil in wok. Stir-fry garlic, carrot and shallot for 1 minute. Add the capsicum and chopped broccoli. Stir-fry for 2-3 minutes or until the vegetables are just tender. Stir through tamari and coriander.
5. Serve 'rice' topped with tofu and sprinkled with seeds and extra shallot and coriander.

Prep: 15 mins

Cook: 20 mins

Total: 35 mins

Servings: 4

Ingredients

- 105g (1/2 cup) French green lentils, rinsed
- 2 baby fennel bulbs, thinly sliced, some fronds reserved
- 130g (1/2 cup) natural yoghurt
- 2 tbsp chopped fresh continental parsley, plus extra parsley leaves, to serve
- 2 tbsp chopped fresh chives
- 1 tbsp chopped fresh tarragon
- 1 tbsp salted baby capers, rinsed, drained
- 1 tsp finely grated lemon rind
- 1/2 red onion, thinly sliced
- 1 tbsp fresh lemon juice

- Pinch of caster sugar
- 60g baby spinach
- 1/2 avocado, sliced
- 180g sliced salt-reduced smoked salmon

Directions

1. Cook lentils in a large saucepan of boiling water for 20 minutes or until tender. Drain.
2. Meanwhile, heat a chargrill pan over high heat. Spray fennel slices with oil. Cook for 2 minutes each side or until tender.
3. Process the yoghurt, parsley, chives, tarragon, capers and lemon rind in a food processor until smooth. Season with pepper.
4. Place onion, juice, sugar and a pinch of salt in a bowl. Set aside for 5 minutes. Drain.
5. Combine the lentils, fennel, onion, spinach and avocado in a large bowl. Divide among plates. Top with salmon. Sprinkle with the reserved fennel fronds and extra parsley. Drizzle with the green goddess dressing.

Prep: 10 mins

Cook: 20 mins

Total: 30 mins

Servings: 4

Ingredients

Vegetables:

- 16 ounces peeled carrots, cut into 1/2" dice to equal about 3 cups
- 8 ounces lightly peeled parsnips, cut into 1/2" dice to equal about 1 1/2 cups
- 8 ounces red potatoes (NOT peeled), cut into 1/2" dice to equal about 1 1/2 cups
- 4 teaspoons extra virgin olive oil
- 1/2 teaspoon kosher salt
- 1/4 teaspoon black pepper

Drizzle:

- 1 1/2 tablespoons apple cider vinegar
- 1 tablespoon extra virgin olive oil
- 1 tablespoon honey
- 1 tablespoon smooth dijon mustard
- 1/16 teaspoon kosher salt
- optional: chopped parsley for garnish

Directions

1. Preheat oven to 475°F. Line a large baking sheet with parchment paper.
2. Toss vegetables with 4 teaspoons oil, 1/2 teaspoon salt, and 1/4 teaspoon black pepper. Make sure that the vegetables are evenly coated with oil, and that the seasonings are distributed throughout. (You can do this in a bowl, or directly on the parchment-lined baking sheet.)
3. Spread the vegetables out on the baking sheet so they aren't piled on top of each other. (If you have a smaller baking sheet and the vegetables are

crowded, it's best to grab a second baking sheet, rather than piling the veggies up.)

4. Roast the vegetables for about 12 minutes. Stir vegetables and continue roasting for 8-10 minutes longer, until the vegetables have toasty, browned, roasted spots but aren't burned.

5. While the vegetables are roasting, whisk together all ingredients for the Honey-Dijon Drizzle (vinegar, olive oil, honey, mustard, and salt).

6. Serve vegetables warm, drizzled with Honey-Dijon sauce and sprinkled with a little chopped fresh parsley, if desired.

Prep: 15 mins

Cook: 20 mins

Total: 35 mins

Servings: 4

Ingredients

- 105g (1/2 cup) French green lentils, rinsed
- 2 baby fennel bulbs, thinly sliced, some fronds reserved
- 130g (1/2 cup) natural yoghurt
- 2 tbsp chopped fresh continental parsley, plus extra parsley leaves, to serve
- 2 tbsp chopped fresh chives
- 1 tbsp chopped fresh tarragon
- 1 tbsp salted baby capers, rinsed, drained
- 1 tsp finely grated lemon rind
- 1/2 red onion, thinly sliced
- 1 tbsp fresh lemon juice

- Pinch of caster sugar
- 60g baby spinach
- 1/2 avocado, sliced
- 180g sliced salt-reduced smoked salmon

Directions

1. Cook lentils in a large saucepan of boiling water for 20 minutes or until tender. Drain.
2. Meanwhile, heat a chargrill pan over high heat. Spray fennel slices with oil. Cook for 2 minutes each side or until tender.
3. Process the yoghurt, parsley, chives, tarragon, capers and lemon rind in a food processor until smooth. Season with pepper.
4. Place onion, juice, sugar and a pinch of salt in a bowl. Set aside for 5 minutes. Drain.
5. Combine the lentils, fennel, onion, spinach and avocado in a large bowl. Divide among plates. Top with salmon. Sprinkle with the reserved fennel fronds and extra parsley. Drizzle with the green goddess dressing.

12. Black Bean Buddha Bowl with Creamy Cashew Dressing

Prep: 20 mins

Cook: 15 mins

Total: 35 mins

Servings: 4

Ingredients

- 200g (1 cup) tri-coloured quinoa, rinsed, drained
- 580ml (2 1/3 cups) water
- 2 tsp ground cumin
- 2 tsp extra virgin olive oil
- 1 red onion, finely chopped
- 2 garlic cloves, crushed
- 2 tsp sweet paprika
- 400g can black beans, rinsed, drained
- 2 zucchini, trimmed, cut into thin noodles
- 2 corncobs, cooked, kernels removed
- Thinly sliced long fresh red chilli, to serve

- Fresh coriander leaves, to serve

- Coriander & cashew dressing

- 50g raw cashews, soaked in cold water for 3 hours

- 1 tbsp lemon juice

- 1 tbsp extra virgin olive oil

- 2 tbsp chopped fresh coriander

- 60ml (1/4 cup) water

Directions

1. Place the quinoa, 2 cups of the water and 1 tsp of the cumin in a saucepan over medium heat. Bring to the boil. Reduce heat to low. Cook, covered for 12 minutes or until the water has been absorbed and the quinoa is al dente.

2. Meanwhile, heat the oil in a saucepan over medium heat. Add the onion. Cook, stirring occasionally, for 5 minutes or until softened. Add the garlic, paprika and remaining cumin. Cook, stirring, for 1 minute or until aromatic. Add the black beans and remaining water. Simmer for 5

minutes or until water has almost evaporated. Coarsely mash the beans with a fork.

3. For the dressing, drain the cashews. Process the cashews, lemon juice, oil and coriander in a small food processor or blender until combined. Gradually add water until thick and creamy.

4. Divide the quinoa, bean mixture, zucchini and corn among bowls. Drizzle with the dressing. Sprinkle with the chilli and coriander.

Prep: 15 mins

Total: 15 mins

Servings: 4

Ingredients

- 1 yellow witlof, leaves separated
- 1 bunch rocket, trimmed
- 3 stalks red kale, leaves chopped
- 125g strawberries, hulled, halved
- 1/4 cup natural almond kernels, toasted
- Strawberry balsamic vinaigrette
- 125g strawberries, hulled, halved
- 2 tbsp grapeseed oil
- 1 tbsp honey
- 3 tsp balsamic vinegar
- 1 tbsp finely chopped fresh basil leaves

Directions

1. Place strawberries, oil, honey and vinegar in a small food processor. Process until smooth. Season with salt and pepper. Stir in basil.
2. Place witlof, rocket, kale, strawberries and almonds on a serving plate. Drizzle with dressing. Serve.

Prep: 30 mins

Cook: 45 mins

Total: 1 hr 15 mins

Servings: 6

Ingredients

- 1kg gold sweet potato, cut crossways into 1cm-thick slices
- 2 tbsp olive oil
- 2 garlic cloves, thinly sliced
- 1/2 cup (50g) walnuts
- 120g pkt Coles Superfood Leaf Blend
- 2 x 250g pkts cooked baby beetroot, quartered
- 1/4 cup (60ml) balsamic dressing

Directions

1. Preheat oven to 200 degrees C. Combine sweet potato, oil and garlic in a roasting pan. Roast for 40 mins or until the sweet potato is tender.

2. Add walnuts and cook for a further 5 mins or until walnuts are toasted. Set aside for 20 mins to cool.

3. Arrange the sweet potato mixture, salad leaves and beetroot on a serving platter. Drizzle with dressing and season.

Prep: 5 mins

Total: 5 mins

Servings: 2

Ingredients

- 25g (1/4 cup) rolled oats
- 2 tbsp The Chia Co black Chia seeds
- 250ml (1 cup) almond milk
- 1/2 tsp ground cinnamon
- 90g (1/3 cup) natural yoghurt
- 1 mango, peeled, sliced
- 2 tbsp natural sliced almonds
- Cinnamon, extra, to serve

Directions

1. Combine the oats and chia seeds in a bowl. Add milk and cinnamon and stir to combine. Cover

with plastic wrap and place in the fridge overnight.

2. Divide the oat mixture between 2 bowls. Top each with yoghurt, mango and almond. Sprinkle with extra cinnamon.

Prep: 20 mins

Cook: 20 mins

Total: 40 mins

Servings: 4

Ingredients

- 1 tsp. ground cumin
- 1/2 tsp. garlic powder
- 1/4 tsp. chipotle chili powder
- kosher salt
- Pepper
- 1 tbsp. olive oil
- 2 large boneless, skinless chicken breasts
- 4 medium radishes
- 2 scallions
- 1 large avocado
- 1/4 c. pomegranate seeds

- 1 tbsp. fresh lime juice

- 1/2 c. fresh cilantro leaves

- 8 small flour tortillas

- sour cream

Directions

1. Heat oven to 425 degrees F. Line a rimmed baking sheet with foil. In a small bowl, combine the cumin, garlic, chili powders, and 1/2 teaspoon salt.

2. Heat the oil in a medium skillet over medium heat. Season the chicken with the spice mixture and cook until browned, 2 to 3 minutes per side. Transfer the chicken to the baking sheet and roast until cooked through, 8 to 10 minutes.

3. Meanwhile, in a medium bowl, gently toss together the radishes, scallions, avocado, pomegranate seeds, lime juice, and 1/4 teaspoon each salt and pepper; fold in the cilantro.

4. Slice the chicken into 1/4-inch-thick pieces. Fill the tortillas with the chicken and top with the

pomegranate salsa. Serve with sour cream, if
desired.

Prep: 5 mins

Cook: 20 mins

Total: 25 mins

Servings: 3

Ingredients

- 400g raw almonds
- 1/4 cup tamari

Directions

1. Preheat oven to 180 degrees C or 160 degress C fan-forced. Line a large baking tray with baking paper.
2. Place almonds on prepared tray. Drizzle over tamari and toss to coat. Arrange in a single layer and bake for 20 minutes, tossing every 5 minutes, or until tamari has evaporated.

3. Cool on tray before storing in an airtight container in a cool dark place.

Prep: 15 mins

Cook: 45 mins

Total: 60 mins

Servings: 4

Ingredients

- 2 tsp extra virgin olive oil
- 1 large red onion, finely chopped
- 3 celery sticks, finely chopped
- 2 garlic cloves, crushed
- 2 tsp finely grated lemon rind
- 1 tsp turmeric
- 1/2 tsp ground cinnamon
- 1/2 tsp dried chilli flakes
- 500ml (2 cups) Massel Vegetable Liquid Stock
- 135g (3/4 cup) French green lentils, rinsed, drained
- 2 vine-ripened tomatoes, chopped

- 150g green beans, trimmed, sliced
- 100g Coles Chopped Kale
- 1 tbsp fresh lemon juice
- 2 tbsp chopped fresh coriander
- Natural yoghurt, to serve (optional)

Directions

1. Heat the olive oil in a large saucepan over medium heat. Add the onion and celery. Cook, stirring occasionally, for 5 minutes or until softened. Add the garlic, lemon rind, turmeric, cinnamon and chilli flakes . Cook, stirring for 1 minute or until aromatic.

2. Add stock, lentils, tomato and 750ml (3 cups) water to the pan. Bring to boil. Reduce the heat to low and partially cover. Simmer for 30 minutes, until lentils are tender.

3. Add the beans and kale to the soup. Stir to combine. Simmer for 3-4 minutes or until the beans are tender-crisp. Stir in the lemon juice and season with pepper. Stir in the coriander just

before serving. Serve topped with a dollop of yoghurt, if you like.

19. Tuna Carpaccio with Grilled Vegies

Prep: 15 mins

Cook: 15 mins

Total: 30 mins

Servings: 4

Ingredients

- 350g tomato medley mix, large ones halved
- 1/4 cup chopped fresh dill
- 2 tsp finely grated lemon rind
- 500g piece sashimi-grade tuna
- 2 tbsp fresh lemon juice
- 1 long fresh red chilli, deseeded, finely chopped
- 1 tbsp salted baby capers, rinsed, drained
- 1 tbsp extra virgin olive oil
- 2 zucchini, thinly sliced lengthways
- 2 bunches asparagus, trimmed
- 1/2 cup small fresh basil leaves

Directions

1. Preheat oven to 160 degrees C/140 degrees C fan forced. Line a baking tray with baking paper.

2. Place the tomatoes on the prepared tray and spray lightly with oil. Bake for 15 minutes, until softened.

3. Meanwhile, combine dill, lemon rind and a pinch of salt on a plate. Roll tuna in the dill mixture to coat. Combine the lemon juice, chilli, capers and olive oil in a small bowl.

4. Heat a chargrill pan over high heat. Spray the zucchini, asparagus and tuna with oil. Cook zucchini and asparagus for 2 minutes each side or until lightly charred and just tender. Cook the tuna for about 1 minute each side or until seared all over.

5. Thinly slice the tuna. Arrange the zucchini, asparagus, tomatoes and basil on serving plates. Top with the sliced tuna and drizzle with the dressing.

Prep: 5 mins

Total: 5 mins

Servings: 2

Ingredients

- 2 large oranges
- 2-inch piece fresh ginger
- 2-inch piece fresh turmeric
- 2 teaspoons vanilla extract
- 2 tablespoons organic maple syrup
- 1/2 teaspoon black pepper
- 2/3 cup organic carrot juice
- 1 cup sparkling water

Directions

1. Zest both oranges and add zest to a high-powered blender. Juice the oranges, adding juice to the blender.

2. Add all remaining ingredients to blender, except the sparkling water. Blend until smooth.

3. Evenly divide turmeric mixture between two large glasses. Top each glass with 1/2 cup sparkling water. Serve and enjoy!

Prep: 10 mins

Total: 10 mins

Servings: 4

Ingredients

- 1/4 cup chopped cilantro
- 2 cloves garlic, minced
- Salt to taste
- 2 ripe avocados, pitted and peeled
- 1/4 cup minced onion
- 2 tbsp minced jalapeño pepper
- Juice of 1 lemon
- 2 oz tortilla chips

Directions

1. Combine the cilantro and garlic on a cutting board and use the back of a chef's knife to work them into a fine paste; a pinch of coarse salt helps

this process. (If you own a mortar and pestle, there's never been a better time to use it.)

2. Transfer the paste to a bowl and add the avocado.

3. Use a fork to mash the avocado into a mostly smooth—but still slightly chunky—purée.

4. Stir in the onion, jalapeño, lemon juice, and salt.

5. Serve with tortilla chips or warm corn tortillas.

Prep: 10 mins

Cook: 25 mins

Total: 35 mins

Servings: 4

Ingredients

- ½ tbsp canola oil
- 1 medium onion, diced
- ½ tbsp minced fresh ginger
- 2 cups cubed butternut squash (Carrots or potatoes would both be perfect substitutes for the squash, just in case butternut is not in season)
- 1 head cauliflower, cut into florets
- 1 can (14–16 oz) garbanzo beans (aka chickpeas), drained
- 1 jalapeño pepper, minced
- 1 tbsp yellow curry powder
- 1 can (14 oz) diced tomatoes

- 1 can (14 oz) light coconut milk
- Juice of 1 lime
- Salt and black pepper to taste
- Chopped cilantro

Directions

1. Heat the oil in a large sauté pan or pot over medium heat.
2. Add the onion and ginger and cook for about 2 minutes, until the onion is soft and translucent.
3. Add the squash, cauliflower, garbanzos, jalapeño, and curry powder. Cook for 2 minutes, until the curry powder is fragrant and coats the vegetables evenly.
4. Stir in the tomatoes and coconut milk and turn the heat down to low.
5. Simmer for 15 to 20 minutes, until the vegetables are tender.
6. Add the lime juice and season with salt and black pepper.
7. Serve garnished with the chopped cilantro.

Prep: 10 mins

Cook: 40 mins

Total: 50 mins

Servings: 4

Ingredients

- ½ tbsp olive oil
- 1 medium carrot, peeled and diced
- ½ medium yellow onion, diced
- 2 cloves garlic, minced
- 1 cup dried lentils
- 3 cups chicken broth or water
- 2 bay leaves
- 2 tbsp red wine vinegar
- Salt and black pepper to taste
- 4 salmon fillets (4 oz each)
- 2 tbsp Dijon mustard
- 2 tbsp brown sugar

Directions

1. Preheat the oven to 450°F.

2. Heat the olive oil in a medium saucepan over medium heat.

3. Add the carrot, onion, and garlic and sauté for 5 to 7 minutes, until soft and lightly browned.

4. Add the lentils, broth, and bay leaves.

5. Simmer for about 20 minutes, until the lentils are tender and the liquid has mostly evaporated.

6. Before serving, add the vinegar, season with salt and pepper, and discard the bay leaves.

7. While the lentils simmer, roast the salmon: Season the fish with salt and black pepper.

8. Combine the mustard and brown sugar in a mixing bowl and spread evenly over the salmon fillets.

9. Place the salmon on a baking sheet and place on the top rack of the oven. Roast for 8 to 10 minutes, until the salmon has browned on the surface and flakes with gentle pressure from your finger.

10. Divide the lentils among 4 plates or pasta bowls and top each serving with a piece of salmon.

Prep: 10 mins

Cook: 10 mins

Total: 20 mins

Servings: 4

Ingredients

- 1 tbsp olive oil
- 3 cloves garlic, thinly sliced
- Pinch red pepper flakes
- 2 bunches spinach, stems removed, washed and dried
- Juice of 1 lemon
- Salt and black pepper to taste

Directions

1. Heat the olive oil in a large sauté or saucepan over medium-low heat.

2. Add the garlic and red pepper flakes and cook gently for about 3 minutes, until the garlic is lightly browned.

3. Add the spinach and cook, moving the uncooked spinach to the bottom of the pan with tongs, for about 5 minutes, until fully wilted.

4. Drain off any excess water from the bottom of the pan.

5. Stir in the lemon juice and season to taste with salt and black pepper.

Prep: 15 mins

Cook: 33 mins

Total: 48 mins

Servings: 4

Ingredients

- 1 large sweet potato, cut into 1/2- to 1-inch cubes
- 1 large apple, cut into similar size cubes as sweet potatoes
- 1 pound Brussels sprouts, trimmed and cut in half
- 6-8 shallots, ends trimmed off, peeled and cut in half (or about the same size as the potatoes)
- 1 pound salmon
- 2/3 cup finely chopped California Walnuts
- 2 tablespoons coarse ground mustard
- 3 tablespoons real maple syrup
- 2 tablespoons olive oil, divided
- 1/2 teaspoon paprika

- 1/4 teaspoon salt more to taste
- 1/4 teaspoon black pepper more to taste

Directions

1. Preheat oven to 425°F.
2. Line a rimmed baking sheet with parchment paper.
3. Toss sweet potatoes, Brussels sprouts, and shallots with 1 tablespoon olive oil (I sometimes do it in a zip-top bag!). Spread on sheet pan and sprinkle with salt and pepper as desired.
4. Place in oven and cook for 15 minutes.
5. Meanwhile, rinse salmon and pat dry. Prepare walnut mixture in a small bowl, stirring together walnuts, mustard, maple syrup, 1 tablespoon olive oil, paprika, salt and pepper.
6. After 15 minutes, toss vegetables around and push them to the edges of the pan to make room for the salmon.

7. Place salmon on pan and spoon walnut mixture on top. Sprinkle apples around the salmon with the vegetables.

8. Return to oven and cook for 15-18 minutes or until fish is flaky or reaches an internal temperature at its thickest portion of 145°F.

Prep: 10 mins

Total: 10 mins

Servings: 12

Ingredients

- 1 1/4 cup rolled oats
- 1/2 cup almond butter
- 1/3 cup maple syrup
- 1/4 cup hemp seeds, shelled
- 1/4 cup shredded coconut, unsweetened
- 1 teaspoon ground turmeric
- 1 teaspoon ground ginger
- 1 teaspoon cinnamon
- 1/4 tsp salt
- 1/8 tsp black pepper

Optional:

- 1-2 tablespoons water, may be needed if mixture is too dry

- 2-3 tablespoons shredded coconut, for rolling, if desired

Directions

1. Combine all ingredients in a food processor and blend until a dough-like consistency is reached. If the mixture is too dry, slowly add 1-2 tablespoons of water.

2. Wet your hands to reduce sticking, and form the batter into 1-inch balls. Don't worry if they aren't holding their shape; they will harden once refrigerated.

3. If desired, pour an extra few tablespoons of shredded coconut onto a plate and roll some or all of the balls for an extra layer of flavor!

4. Lay balls onto a baking sheet lined with parchment paper and place in refrigerator for at least two hours to harden.

5. Store in an airtight container in the refrigerator or freezer, and enjoy!

Prep: 10 mins

Cook: 20 mins

Total: 30 mins

Servings: 4

Ingredients

- Nonstick cooking spray
- 12 oz sweet potato, scrubbed and cut into 1/2-inch pieces
- 1 medium red or yellow onion, sliced into wedges
- 4 tbsp olive oil
- 1 tsp salt
- 1/2 tsp black pepper
- 1/4 tsp ground cinnamon
- 2 tbsp rice wine vinegar
- 1 tbsp curry powder
- 2 tsp honey
- 1/2 tsp salt

- 1/4 tsp black pepper
- 2 cups cooked wild rice
- 4 oz cooked chicken, shredded
- 1/4 cup golden or regular raisins
- 2 medium carrots, shaved
- 1/4 cup snipped fresh cilantro

Directions

1. Preheat oven to 400°F. Line a baking sheet with foil, and coat with cooking spray.
2. In a medium bowl, combine sweet potato, onion, 1 tbsp oil, 1/2 tsp salt, 1/4 tsp pepper, and cinnamon; toss to coat. Transfer potato mixture to prepared baking sheet. Roast about 20 minutes or until tender.
3. Meanwhile, in a small bowl, combine remaining 3 tbsp oil, vinegar, curry powder, honey, the remaining 1/2 tsp salt, and the remaining 1/4 tsp pepper. Whisk until smooth.
4. Divide rice among four pint jars. Top with roasted potatoes, chicken, raisins, and carrots. Drizzle

with dressing and top with cilantro. Cover and
chill up to 3 days.

Prep: 20 mins

Additional: 1 hr 40 mins

Total: 2 hrs

Servings: 4

Ingredients

- 1 qt. vanilla yogurt
- 1 tbsp. coriander seeds
- 1 tsp. cumin seeds
- 1/2 tsp. black peppercorns
- 1 tsp. fennel seeds
- 1 tsp. turmeric
- 1/2 tsp. mustard seed
- 1/2 tsp. ginger
- 2 c. raw mixed nuts
- 1/4 c. corn syrup
- 1 tsp. orange zest
- 1 tsp. Sea salt

- 2 c. blueberries or cherries

- 1/4 c. sugar

Directions

1. Place yogurt in the bowl of an ice cream maker; process according to the manufacturer's instructions, then freeze 1 hour to fully solidify.

2. Meanwhile, combine whole spices in a medium skillet over medium-low heat. Cook, shaking often for 2 to 3 minutes. Transfer to a bowl to cool completely, then grind to a fine powder using a spice grinder or a mortar and pestle. Add remaining spices, and mix well.

3. Preheat oven to 350 degrees F, and line 2 baking sheets with parchment paper. Place nuts in a medium bowl. Add corn syrup; toss well to coat. Mix in ground spices, orange zest, and sea salt; toss to evenly coat nuts. Spread nuts on baking sheets, and roast in oven until corn syrup is bubbly, 15 to 20 minutes. Cool completely.

4. Meanwhile, make a fruit sauce by combining berries, sugar, and 1/2 cup water in a saucepan over low heat. Bring to a simmer; cook, stirring occasionally, about 15 minutes. Cool completely.

5. To serve, scoop frozen yogurt into 4 bowls; top each with nuts and sauce.

Prep: 20 mins

Cook: 30 mins

Total: 50 mins

Servings: 4

Ingredients

- 2 cloves garlic, minced
- 1 tbsp finely chopped fresh rosemary (Almost any herb works here: thyme, parsley, oregano, basil, or sage)
- Zest and juice of 1 lemon
- 1 tbsp olive oil
- 1 chicken (4 lb)
- Salt and black pepper to taste
- 1 large russet potato, sliced into 1/8" rounds
- 2 onions, quartered
- 4 large carrots, cut into large chunks

Directions

1. Preheat the oven to 450°F. Mix the garlic, rosemary, lemon zest, and half of the olive oil.

2. Working on the chicken, gently separate the skin from the flesh at the bottom of the breast and spoon in half of the rosemary mixture; use your hands to spread it around as thoroughly as possible.

3. Spread the remaining half over the top of the chicken and then season with plenty of salt and pepper.

4. Mix the potato, onions, carrots, remaining olive oil, and a good pinch of salt and pepper.

5. Arrange the vegetables in the bottom of a roasting pan and place the chicken on top, breast side up.

6. Roast for 20 to 30 minutes, until the skin is lightly browned.

7. Reduce the oven temperature to 350°F and roast for another 30 minutes or so.

8. The chicken is done when the juices between the breast and the leg run clear and an instant-read

thermometer inserted deep into the thigh reads 155°F.

9. Remove from the oven and allow to rest for 10 minutes before carving.

10. Serve with the vegetables.

Prep: 10 mins

Cook: 10 mins

Total: 20 mins

Servings: 4

Ingredients

- 1 head of cauliflower
- 1 tbsp olive oil
- 2 garlic cloves, minced
- 1-2 tsp finely chopped herbs, thyme, rosemary, sage, parsley, chives, etc

Directions

1. Trim the leaves off the cauliflower and cut off the florets. Rinse the florets under water.
2. Heat 1-inch of water in a pot on medium heat and bring to a boil. Place a steamer insert in the pot

and add the cauliflower florets. Steam for 6-8 minutes.

3. While the cauliflower is steaming, heat the olive oil in a small pan on medium heat. Add the minced garlic and cook for 30 seconds, then remove from the heat.

4. Remove the steamed cauliflower from the pot, drain the water from the pot, then add the cauliflower back in. Add the olive oil, garlic, chopped herbs and any optional ingredients.

5. Use a potato masher or handheld stick blender to mash the cauliflower. Serve immediately.